MEENA KUMARI

Introduction to Yoga
What Yoga Means?
Learn Different Paths of Yoga
Methods of Shatkarma
What Yoga Offers?

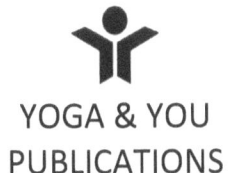

YOGA & YOU
PUBLICATIONS

Preface

It is a remarkable time nowadays that a keen interest in yoga is developing among the educated and intellectuals in most of the countries. Health is the basis of a happy and prosperous life. The first and foremost principle for healthy living is the prevention of diseases.

Man is mortal and death is inevitable. It is the innate instinctive nature of living creatures to sustain life and postpone death. The lowest creatures which roam about freely in the natural surroundings eat whatever they get and seldom fall sick.

Whenever a man breaks the law of nature, there is an imbalance between the following five elements, the disease comes making the body lifeless:

1. Akash (*Sky*)
2. Vayu (*Air*)
3. Agni (*Fire*)
4. Jal (*Water*)
5. Prithvi (*Earth*)

The one, who keeps the proper balance of these five elements, seldom falls sick. There are more cases of mental imbalance and psychic disorders than other diseases.

Yoga is not a religion; it is the search for inner development of the consciousness, going directly to the very heart of reality. It does not involve simply obeying traditional rules or following well-established modes of social and cultural behavior. It is a way of progressively realizing one's full potential thus arriving at the complete emancipation of the mind.

Yoga is the gift of the ancient sages and savants of India. It is a treasure from which physical, mental, social and spiritual benefits accrue.

My first book "Yoga for Health and Happiness" provides a ready reference about asanas and pranayama which are well chosen and expertly described. The language is simple and apt. I am sure the public at large will be benefited by this book.

May yoga prosper well and bring happiness to the world.

MEENA KUMARI
M.A., LLB., P.G. Dip.
In Public Relations and French,
N.D.D.Y.

DEDICATION

This book is dedicated to my Guru, Late Swami Anandanand
(25th January 1902 – 19th June 1991).

Table of Contents

"When the mind and body are working together harmoniously due to yoga discipline, we can find calm and peace at every moment."

- *Bhagavad Gita*

"The self cannot be known by one, who is dull or restless, who is not strong, disciplined and self-controlled. Neither can it be known by much learning nor by reasoning. It can be known only through calmness of mind, through the practice of yoga and through meditation."

- *Upanishad*

"Mastery of the body and breath are an undoubted aid to those concerned with their spiritual evolution. For by having full control over the physical condition, the body becomes calm, allowing the mind to be directed inwardly more easily in perfect tranquility to achieve a higher spiritual level."

- *Hatha Yoga Pradipika*

"There is no limit to the power of human mind. The more concentrated it is, the more power is brought to bear on one point. The powers of the mind are like rays of light dissipated, when they are concentrated they illumine."

-   *Swami Vivekananda*

Chapter 1:

INTRODUCTION

INTRODUCTION

The human body is an integrated whole of five elements. Whenever there is an imbalance in these elements the disease comes. A human being is a Part and Parcel of nature. As Sun, water, ether, air, and earth are present in the whole world, similarly there is the prominence of these elements in the human body.

A man cannot survive long if he stays away from nature. Though the body is made up of different systems, each system influences the work of the other system and is simultaneously influenced by them. The blood, for instance, in the course of its unceasing circulation carries materials to the various parts of the body and supplies them living tissues as well as oxygen which is so essential for life.

The heart, the lungs, the brain, will at once stop functioning if the blood circulation stops for a moment. But it is the heart which pumps up blood and keeps it in circulation while the lungs supply it with oxygen and remove carbon dioxide from it. The harder a muscle is worked, the greater is its need of oxygen and nutritive material. By regular work, a muscle not only strengthens itself but also intensifies the activity of the organs of respiration and blood circulation and in this way exercises the muscles of the throat and heart.

Besides this, exercise increases appetite arouses a feeling of general vigor and as a result, the vital activity of the whole organism is increased. The muscular effort also influences the bones. It helps in developing ridges on which the muscles can be firmly attached, and then the activities of the muscles are also responsible for the proper development of the bones.

Thus all systems depend upon one another for maintaining the normal functions of the human body.

Human physiology is the study of the functions of the human body, of the life activities of the organs and the organism as a whole. Likewise, to understand the structure of the organs of the body, it is necessary to have a correct understanding of their functions. Any change in the function of an organ results in the change of its structure, and vice versa. For example, all the muscles which are properly exercised become stronger and increase in size, but the muscles which are not worked often, are enfeebled and start weakening. Thus maintaining all the muscles of the body in the fit fettle, they have all to be properly exercised. And Yoga is perhaps the only system of exercise which can work up all the muscles and thus have an all-round effect.

Muscular work usually requires sustained effort on the part of the organism but when the effort is combined with pleasure, the organism can do the work without minding strain of the hard work. Yoga exercises combine pleasure with muscular work.

Exercises help to strengthen the muscles of the heart. The degree to which one can do hard physical work depends upon one's age and physical condition. Naturally, a younger person in good health can do a greater amount of physical work than an aged man or a young man with weak physique.

Chapter 2:

WHAT YOGA MEANS

WHAT YOGA MEANS

Yoga is an invaluable treasure of Bharatiya (Indian) culture. Ancient Indian saints and seers developed it during the past several years. Yoga is the bridge for the union of the Jeevatma and Paramatma.

Yoga is so ancient that we have no definite knowledge of its origin. We find its mention in the Vedas, which was created some 2,500 years before Christ. Yet figures of yogic *asanas* in meditation have been traced in rock paintings from times even earlier than the Vedic period. There is mention of the meditational yoga even in the pre-Aryan culture but there is no mention anywhere of its practical aspect, which must have come later with the Yogis having to find easy and effective exercises to work their cramped muscles after sitting for a long period in meditational postures. Thus Yoga is developed into a complete system of self-culture to strengthen body and mind. Yoga has also been described as skillful living amongst activities or wisdom of work, moderation, and harmony.

Word Yoga is derived from Sanskrit root 'Yuj' to unite or to combine with Supreme Being. Yoga means discipline of the mind and body. The absolute aspect of sex and health lies in yoga and it provides a spiritual yet radiant outlook on life. One might choose its physical, scientific and spiritual aspect according to one's approach towards yoga.

Yoga is neither acrobatics nor mere physical fitness but an all-round beneficial system to provide both physical and spiritual health. The practice of yoga is not meant just for the benefit of the physically weak or psychologically imbalanced but more so for the smooth running and efficient working of the psychosomatic machine.

One of the greatest benefits of yoga lies in its potential to strengthen the nervous system which is controller and coordinator of all the systems in the human body. Through the practice of yoga, the restless mind is calmed down and energy is diverted from the destructive in constructive channels.

The mind is restless and hard to control. Mind causes pain and agony by its unbridled acts. Yoga helps in controlling the waywardness of mind and thereby destroying all pains and sorrows and bringing peace and harmony of mind.

Chapter 3:

DIFFERENT PATHS OF YOGA

DIFFERENT PATHS OF YOGA

Yoga means union, union of man's individual spirit with the spirit of the universe or God. However, there is more than one method of achieving this union. But all the methods lead to the same goal. Though each of these yogic paths is distinguished by its particular practice, they cannot be rigidly classified or put into watertight compartments. They overlap, merge and become diffused at certain points of training. Spiritual enlightenment is not dependent on intellect or education. Although scholars and men of great mental gifts are more drawn to yoga, there is something above intellect, a direct channel to divinity which makes a person suitable for yoga practice. By understanding that all systems of yoga lead to the same final goal, we can go deep into any of the systems depending on our capabilities and inclinations.

Some of the different paths of yoga are as follows:

1. Hatha Yoga
2. Karma Yoga
3. Bhakti Yoga
4. Jnana Yoga
5. Raja Yoga
6. Kundalini Yoga

1.   Hatha Yoga

Cleanliness of the body is the declared objective of Hatha yoga. Every living being aspires for the longevity of life by keeping the body healthy.

According to ancient Sanskrit facts, 'Ha' means the sun or the Pingala Nadi, which works on the right, 'Tha' signifies the moon or the Chandra Nadi which flows on the left. To inhale is the 'Ha' and to exhale is the 'Tha'.

Hatha yoga is the path of bodily strength and control. Liberation through Hatha yoga involves bringing the body to its highest state of development and under complete control of the mind.

For Hatha yoga, concentration and identification is a must. Concentration is the total attention kept focused at one point because it brings power to still the mind.

Identification is the state of extreme concentration that the personality becomes merged with the object of contemplation. Identification leads to the liberation of the spirit, and one feels united with God.

2. Karma Yoga

No person can keep himself away from 'Karma' (action). Man is a social animal. Humanity is the most precious jewel he possesses but being swayed by temptations and blinded by selfishness he leads to sinful acts. Doing everything in life with the fullest and utmost love of God is Karma yoga.

Remaining unconcerned about the fruit of the actions done, fulfilling family obligations and social demand, to live in complete harmony with the humanity is Karma yoga.

Karma yoga is the path of the right action. This is a practical path for men and women who must lead an active life as householders in a materialistic society.

It does not require withdrawal from the world nor impose any rigid training. It is the path of duty and right action.

The Karmayogi works as hard as he can and enjoys the material fruits of his work but at heart, he remains detached and free from worldly affairs.

3. Bhakti Yoga

The essence of yoga sadhana (*practice*) consists in the sadhaka's filling himself to the brim. i.e. fully with God's boundless power, vast endless knowledge, limitless love and immense joy.

Attachment, lust, vanity, temptation are the real obstacles in the path of Sadhaka (*seeker*). To reach the Bhakti stage, faith (Shraddha), confidence (Nishta), and devotion (Bhakti) are very necessary.

Bhakti yoga is the path of devotion. The yoga of love and devotion always appeals to those who live more by emotions than by intellect.

This is the most popular yoga among the people of India, for it makes no great intellectual demands and requires no special training.

Bhakti yoga appeals to man's instinctive nature and recognizes the love of all kinds as a form of worship, whether lovers, parents, children or friends.

4.   Jnana Yoga

Knowledge is endless and boundless. Following the developmental changes and realizing the greatness of the creation and reposing oneself with the seat of parmabrama to meditate on it is called Jnana yoga.

A sadhaka developing his discrimination (veiveka) absence of worldly desires and temptations (Vairagya), starving after final emancipation moves near his deliverance (Mukti).

Jnana yoga, the path of knowledge, attracts intellectuals and philosophers, those who must know the reason behind everything, the secrets of creation.

It is a difficult and lonely path for its demands are too great for the average man.

The Jnana Yogi steps aside from life and dedicates himself to find truth through the highest form of thought.

He is withdrawn and detached from society and has his own personality.

5. Raja Yoga

In Raja yoga, greater importance is given to pranayama, Along with Pooraka, Kumbhaka, and Rechaka, the sadhaka is to destroy all dualism and secure control over the powers of the world.

Pranayama is of great help in achieving excellence in Dharana, Dhyana and Samadhi the sure ways of bringing external forces under one's control is to control one's mind.

"Yogas Chitta Vriti Nirodha" i.e. controlling the tendencies of one's reasoning mind is called yoga according to Rishi Patanjali.

Raja yoga brings complete mastery of the mind. It is connected with the attainment of full power and control of the mind.

Raja Yoga, the highest or the King of yoga is often described as the last stage of development and like the Jnana yoga is for the few rather than the majority.

Raja yoga is concerned with the attainment of full power and control of the mind. It is the yoga of wisdom, balance, control, and emergence.

6.   Kundalini Yoga

Kundalini which resides in a dormant state in the upper part of a root is for the attainment of Moksha for the yogis.

The three Nadis (Ida, Pingala, and Sushumna) and six chakras (Mooldhara, Swadhisthana, Manipura, Anahata, Vishudha and Ajna) are related to Kundalini.

The six glands located in the Sushumna Nadi (between Mooldhara and Brahmrandhara) are called Shatchakra.

Arousing the Mooldhara based dormant Kundalini (Shayita-Supta) by yogic Kriya (exercises) and making it flow by Sushumna Nadi via the above Shatchakras and reach the Brahmrandhra is known as arousing the Kundalini.

Kundalini Yoga is the development of mysterious energies of the body. Kundalini is stated to be a "coiled serpent lying dormant at the base of the spine" and when it is aroused through appropriate practices; it uncoils and springs up, hissing through the spine to the top of the brain.

The ultimate purpose of the yoga is to awaken the Kundalini which has been defined as the cosmic power underlying all organic and inorganic matters within us. A yogi who has controlled Kundalini can achieve Samadhi at will.

Whatever path a true yogi follows, he is always striving for an objective where the barrier of mind and body fall away and permit him to liberate his spirit.

Chapter 4:

METHODS OF SHATKARMA

METHODS OF SHATKARMA

A healthy body is of great importance for success in all walks of life. The pioneers in Hatha yoga have prescribed Shatkarma by which one can not only keep illness away but also cure it.

Shatkarma is divided into the following six:

1. Gajakarnee
2. Dhauti
3. Neti
4. Nauli
5. Kapala Bhatee
6. Bhastrika

Bhagee, Bastee, Shankhaprakshalana, and Tratka are also added in Shatkarma later on.

Next, I will explain these different methods and benefits of Shatkarma in more detail for your better understanding.

1.   Gajakarnee

Method:

Sitting in Kagasana pose, drink at least 2 liters of warm water and then bending forward make an angle of 90° with the rest of the body.

Place left hand below the navel. Place three middle fingers of the right hand in the mouth and move them round and round touching the uvula.

This will make all the water flow out to keep on repeating.

Benefits:

It is highly beneficial in stomach disorders like indigestion, gastric trouble, obesity etc.

2.   Dhauti aka *Dhautee*

Method:

Take a piece of 'Mulmul', 24" long and 4" wide. Fully drench it in hot water and swallow it gradually and slowly and pull it out slowly.

Benefits:

It is highly effective in treating cold, cough, asthma and other respiratory diseases.

3.   Neti

Method:

(a) **Sootra Neti**:

This is a 9" long and 1/10" thick thread or slender string divided into two parts. One part is twisted and the rest is untwisted. Dip this in warm rock-salt solution. Sitting in Kagasana pose, put the twisted end of the neti or string in one nostril and get it (the end) out of the mouth slowly. Hold the two ends of the string and move them up and down. Repeat the process with the other nostril.

(b) **Jala Neti**:

This exercise needs a 'Lota', a spherical vessel with a narrow spout. Dissolve rock-salt in warm water held in the lota. Sitting in Kagasana pose and leaning slightly forward, place the spout to the nostril in such a way that the water flows into one nostril and comes out of the other. Repeat the operation with another nostril.

Benefits:

This exercise improves eyesight and is an effective treatment for cold, asthma, bleeding from the nose, headache, mental disorders, forgetfulness, etc.

4. Nauli

Method:

Take a standing position, Bend at the waist and placing palms on knees, bring out Nauli (abdomen) and rotate it. Do for twenty times.

Benefits:

This is highly beneficial to persons suffering from digestive trouble, obesity, indigestion, etc.

5.   Kapala Bhati

Method:

After having done Sootra neti and Jala neti stand up, bend forward at an angle of 90° at the waist and placing hands at the back of the waist and rapidly moving the head in circles, very quietly do the inhaling and exhaling as if you are sneezing. The action will draw out all water in the nose. Repeat the operation at least a hundred times.

Benefits:

The action will draw out all water in the nose. Repeat the operation at least a hundred times.

6. Bhastrika

Method:

Taking Padmasana pose and placing the left palm near the navel, close one nostril with the thumb of the right hand and quickly exhale through the other nostril. Repeat the exercise changing the order of nostrils used and repeat fifty times.

Benefits:

Though this exercise comes under Pranayama, it is given here for the specific purpose of draining the last drops of water from the nostril after Kapala Bhati exercise. It is good for cold, cough and headache.

Chapter 5:

WHAT YOGA OFFERS

WHAT YOGA OFFERS

Through yoga elevation and meditation techniques, one can gain a better emotional control and tranquilize one's agitated and disturbed mind. The best meal and the best tonics are of no avail if one is mentally disturbed. Yoga alone can help in such cases and rectify the defect. Yoga is unbounded by time and space. It helps us to survive physically and psychologically. The primary aim of yoga is to develop through gradual stages, a quality of mind, which can perceive reality and acquire self-confidence through the healthy functioning of the mind and emotions.

Regardless of age, a great number of people of India as well as in the west have started performing yoga exercises because yoga not only attunes the body and mind but also provides a balanced exercise to all parts of the body thus adding beauty and charm to one's personality. It helps one to develop into a well-integrated human being. One can derive immense benefits from its rational systems of exercises and breathing techniques. The very object of asanas is to provide well-being and stability.

Yoga if practiced without break can prove of immense value. Yoga is a means to get rid of stiffness, aches, pains, anxiety neurosis excitements, and depression. Yoga exercises have certain superiority over sex. It is a builder of great sexual stability between marriage partners. Yoga can establish a stable, permanent association based on mutual affection and affectionate companionship.

Sex is the key to good health and health is the key to good sex but yoga is the key to good health as well as good sex. Yoga postures if done correctly, aim at nervous control and purification and increase the health and strength of the internal organs.

The special significance of yoga is that it does not conceive you as having only a physical body but emphasizes the great value of the mind which characterizes your personality. It should be remembered that it not only refers to good health but includes the physical, mental and moral psychic health as well. Good health is your natural privilege and it is easy to be healthy than to be sick.

The aim of daily yoga exercises is not only to acquire a healthy body but it has a direct bearing on the nervous system. Yoga claims that even behavior, character and personality of an individual could either be completely transformed or be adjusted to harmony with social life and moral ideals. It helps to avoid diseases and is an assurance to positive health.

All yoga exercises are of endurance where each movement is within one's own power. So the special feature and importance of the yoga exercises and their dynamic variation lie not only in their peculiar combinations and varieties of physical movement but also the adjustments and choice of breath and respiratory stand and the still and full attention of the mind. In yoga, the physical body merely serves as an instrument of education for the mind and the nervous system which is of paramount importance.

Could You Help?

I'd love to hear your opinion about my book. In the world of book publishing, there are few things more valuable than honest reviews from a wide variety of readers.

Your review will help other readers find out whether my book is for them. It will also help me reach more readers by increasing the visibility of my book.

You can leave your review on Amazon.com.

www.ingramcontent.com/pod-product-compliance
Lightning Source LLC
Chambersburg PA
CBHW050526290526
45786CB00007B/2708